# 3691 Healthy Eating System
# Eat - Move - Live
# And Love It

*Simple Recipes that took me from Out of Shape to Ironman*

**On Average we habitually eat only:**

3 different breakfasts 6 different lunches 9 different dinners and habitually crave 1 particular sweet treat almost daily.

Everybody has their own 3-6-9-1... Inside this book you'll see mine and how changing it, Changed my life!

And how, with the help of my husband, I went from an out of shape, hypoglycemic, couldn't jog around the block without gasping for air kind of girl to an Ironman triathlete. These are the recipes and eating style that I incorporate today and it's 180 degrees different from what I used to eat. Your 3-6-9-1 is creating the current body you reside in... Ready to change it? Take a look at what the 3-6-9-1 system can do for you...

**See the rest of our series:**

3-6-9-1 For Runners
3-6-9-1 Goes Raw
3-6-9-1 on a Budget

3-6-9-1 for Vegetarians
3-6-9-1 on the Go!
3-6-9-1 for the Fitness Enthusiast

Think you have a Super healthy 3-6-9-1 you'd like to share with the world?
Email us.... we'd love to see it and get you in the next book of the series!
staff@Eat3691.com

## Disclaimer

The information presented is not intended for the treatment or prevention of disease, nor is it a substitute for medical treatment, nor as an alternative to medical advice. This publication is presented for information purposes, to increase the public knowledge of developments in the field of strength and conditioning. The program outlined herein should not be adopted without a consultation with your health professional. Use of the information provided is at the sole choice and risk of the reader. You must get your physician's approval before beginning this or any other exercise or nutrition program. This information is not a prescription. Consult your doctor, nutritionist or dietician for further information. The author and the publisher assume no responsibility for any actions of the reader as a result of applying these methods.

# Table of Contents

Eat3691.com

# Getting started with the 3-6-9-1 System

As a fitness, and nutrition, expert I get asked all the time "What do *you* eat to get that body?" that led us to putting together a series of recipe books based on exactly that..."What We Eat".

Have you ever wanted to be a fly on the wall and see exactly what your trainer, or friend with that amazing body, or athlete you look up to, eats like, lives like, moves like?

That's part of what we're sharing with you here in this book. We sculpt our bodies and our lives by what we eat and how much we move. Eat like us, move like us, and you will perform and look like us.

 80% of the way you look and feel is attributed to what you put in your mouth. What you eat is that important! As we researched our clients diets we find a theme. There isn't as much variety as we *think* we have in our diets. We all tend to be creatures of habit and if those habits don't change neither will our health or weight.

One of the most common mistakes we see clients make, before coming to us, is in trying to search out *hidden* culprits in their diets. Like CSI detectives they desperately try to find and blame little things like, the Hershey's kiss they sneak off the desk, every day, or the creamer they put in their coffee.

Confused dieters search their diets looking for a criminal, when the culprit is standing right in front of them, like the elephant in the room, It's their 3-6-9!

When we sit down and *really* look at our clients "go to" staple meals (not what they think they eat but what they habitually gravitate to each week) we see the problem immediately.

What we think we eat, those healthy meals we tell ourselves we get really don't happen all that frequently, or it's one in a long list of poor choices.

When you take the emotion and excuses (I'm too busy) out of the equation and look instead, as an objective observer at what you eat, the most often, you'll find a pattern...

By looking at your diet in this way and removing one or two of the least healthy meals from the rotation and adding just one or two healthier meals you will have made a ten percent difference in your diet and 10% is a lot!

Find more than one or two new meals, you like, and are willing to make staples in your diet and you will begin to see the effects immediately...without it feeling like work!

Yes the best part is when you find meals you really like none of this will seem like a diet or a struggle and you will have made healthy changes without feeling like you had to *force* anything.

All we're asking you to do is LOVE what you eat...

The key to success with the 3,6,9,1 series, and what separates it from all the other diets out there; we are addressing the meals in your life that are habitual. We are asking you to consciously take a moment and take a look at your "go to" meals and put a new meal in the line up...

A new meal that's
- Just as tasty
- Just as easy to make
- and just as comforting

What better way to find great tasting, healthy, "go to" meals than by going to the source and asking health and fitness experts "Hey what do you eat every day to look that way?" In this series, we have scoured the globe and come back with precisely that answer... The favorite things the healthiest people around the world eat, the most often. This is the concept behind the 3,6,9,1 series and we look forward to sharing what this system can do for you!

First of all it can <u>and will</u> transform your body. I know because it did mine... which leads us to our next chapter... Baby I was not born this way!

# Baby I was NOT born this way!

Today I am the owner of a successful health and fitness company, author and athlete. Today I have completed countless races; 5k's, 10k's, half marathons, Marathons, Ironman triathlons, adventure races, walked the 500 mile Camino de Santiago...

But baby I didn't used to be anything like this and that's my main reason for starting this series. Because from where I sit I know there is nothing that separates you from me. I am not special. All of the experts in our 3-6-9-1 series are not special... you can achieve all that we do and more. You can transform your body just as we have.

I eat and move differently than you do now... If you take the steps to make the changes your body will change too.

A brief history... I think it's easy sometimes to blow off your trainers and assume "We were always this way"... Right? It's easy to look at my body and think "well she's just super athletic naturally". "They're just natural athletes" but the truth of the matter is if you believe those things you are doing yourself a horrible disservice because you are excusing yourself out of achieving what you're truly capable of...We weren't always this way... None of us!

The first memory I have of running (as in for sport) is PE class in high school. I was mortified in PE Class because my legs were so fat and they made us change into these really short shorts for class. I HATED that class! The sad thing was I liked moving, I liked the games, I wanted to play. I even liked my coaches but the shorts made me want to break down in tears every day in the locker room and so that would taint the rest of the activities. I was just so uncomfortable and embarrassed and took my fair share of taunting from my friends and classmates but quite literally most of the damage was done by me and my own thoughts. So anyway needless to say I wasn't the star athlete in the class.

And then when it came to running I was the worst! Literally I'm pretty sure I was the last to come in every time we had to run a lap. So when mile run day came... I would try my best and usually come in gasping, ready to throw up or just not complete it at all.

Eat3691.com

I was pear shaped and ashamed of my body. Told it was genetics "Oh you've got those Italian hips" and for years, all the way into young adulthood, I believed it. I believed wholeheartedly that I was just cursed with fat legs and a big butt.

Then slowly, but surely, with the help of my husband I began to learn about nutrition, exercise, endurance, strength training, discipline and consistency and slowly, but surely, my body that I was convinced I was stuck with for life.. began to transform...

My wish for every client of mine and every person who reads this book and the continuing 3-6-9 series is that you begin to believe in the power of your body to transform. Whether you're looking to heal an illness, live a longer more vibrant life, reshape your body, excel at sports or all of the above... My wish for you is that you begin to see how amazing your body really is and that it is possible! Eat like us, move like us and you will live like us!

Welcome to my 3-6-9-1...

Eat3691.com

## Putting the 3-6-9-1 system to work for you...

What we're sharing with you here is our 3,6,9,1. The meals we eat the most often. We are not trying to "blow your mind" with exquisite recipes and beautiful plates. We're simply showing you what we do, on day to day basis. Our most common meals which give us the body and activity levels we desire.

A common mistake we see people make is in not making the UNBELIEVABLY important connection that what you eat is creating the way your body; looks, feels, heals and performs. What you eat is everything... But not only what you eat but *how you feel* about what you eat. This makes your emotional relationship to food of extreme importance! If you're telling yourself you are on a diet. It won't work because the very word conjures up negative emotional feelings; lacking, restricted, "not allowed", deprived... In fact how you feel about what you eat effects how your body processes what you eat. The meaning you give to the foods you eat are what we call the "stories" you tell yourself about food. Look if there was no emotional connection, to food, you would have absolutely no problem adhering to a diet. We go into more depth about this "relationship" to food in our book *Its Not about the Scale* but here we just want to underline the importance of understanding... What you eat, and the "stories" you tell about your 3-6-9-1, is giving you the body you sit in right now. If you want that to change you've got to take a clear cut look at what you're eating habitually and create new "stories" for yourself about what food means.

### 3-6-9-1 is about finding new habitual meals, you are in LOVE with, and ultimately never dieting again!

So to start here's what you'll want to do... Take the time, right now, to read the next couple pages and really think about what you eat the most often. The more real you can be with yourself the more of an effect the 3-6-9-1 system will have for you... Read on and let's get started.

## Write down your 3,6,9,1

Take a moment and write down the breakfasts you eat the most often… It's important, in this step, that your really honest with yourself.

Just ask yourself "what did I eat this morning".. Yesterday". So often we tell ourselves we eat healthy, all the time, but when we really look back over the facts, cut and dry, black and white what we really eat is different than what we think we eat.

So jot down the three breakfast meals you gravitate towards the most often, if you're like most people it looks something like this:

#1 Coffee or beverage (a.k.a. didn't eat at all)
#2 muffin or pastry
#3 egg dish or cereal

Great did you get it written down?

Now do the same with what you generally eat for lunch and then move onto dinner…

When you're finished with this task you will probably find it falls in the ball park of the average

3 breakfast choices, 6 lunches and 9 dinners. If not don't worry this isn't a test.. The main thing here is just to bring attention to the fact that for the vast majority of us there are meals we kind of always have in the line up. Our "go to" meals and if we can switch some of those out and create some new habit patterns we will make a big effect on our waistline and our health!

Eat3691.com

## Step Two

Now that you have your line up clearly in front of you let's start looking at what we definitely want to keep and which ones we could care less about. We just eat them because they're handy or it's habit.

Pizza on that list? Fast food?

Rate them in priority of how much you really enjoy that food.. what you're really getting out of that food experience

- Socially (is there always pizza on bowling night?)
- economically (do you eat it because it's cheap)
- convenience (eat it because there's no time)
- nutrition wise
- familiarity (just because you've always eaten it)
- Yummy factor (it's just darn good)

As you rate your meals you will want to look for replacements which fall into the same category. For example if a meal is a "go to" meal for you because it's inexpensive, choose a new 3,6,9 that meets that requirement. You want to honor what was initially being met with your original meal. If it was a socially fun meal to eat make sure you search our 3,6,9 for a meal that will be fun as well.

What are you basing your rating system on?

Now rate it based on Nutrition only

And come up with the healthiest ...Our definition of the healthiest is simple "Real Food" if possible no tin, no package, no processed etc.....

Everybody's 3-6-9-1 can be made to be healthier without any effort or changing the meal. Let's look at the bottom 5 meals and how to ditch those (get new ones) or change them (the ingredients or how they are made) in other words do we have a similar dish that's made a little healthier than how you are currently making it?

## Step 3 Pay attention to Nutrition labels

In order to be healthy you have to know what it is you're putting in your mouth. For instance did you know that "natural vanilla or raspberry flavor" can be a code word for Castoreum which is…..You might want to sit down for this one (seriously) the secretions from the anal glands of a beaver? Yes the word "Natural" is one of the most dangerous words on our food labels because it gives you a false sense of security, that what you're about to eat is safe, which couldn't't be further from the truth!

When it comes to reading labels, first of all, try to eat as many things that don't have a label as possible. When was the last time you saw a head of broccoli with a nutrition label on it?

Second flip the package over…….The front of the package was designed to do one thing lie to you, sell to you and get you to buy it…. not to inform you. They will say anything possible to get you to purchase the item and that's what the front of the package is for so FLIP IT OVER and read the back. Read the list of ingredients. If you don't understand what the items are YOU SHOULDN'T BE PUTTING IT IN YOUR MOUTH OR YOUR KIDS!

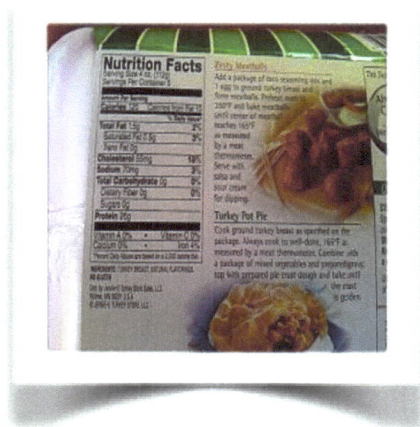

What happens when it comes in a package and it's a main staple in your diet that can't be avoided? Here are two of the most common pitfalls we see people fall into: "choosing the right Ground Turkey" and "making a healthy choice when it comes to spaghetti sauce". So here we go.

Many of the recipes you see below call for "Ground Turkey". If you are trying to cut back on saturated fats it's very important that you purchase the "correct" turkey because most ground turkey you find in stores (and restaurants) is over 50% fat because they grind up and use all parts of the turkey not just breast meat.

When you see "Ground turkey" used in the recipes below we are referring to Turkey breast meat only. Here is an example of what the nutrition label for turkey breast will look like....around 10% fat. You can determine how much fat is in the item by looking at the nutrition label and calculating the total number of calories and the calories from fat.

That will tell you what percentage of fat the item is actually made up of (as opposed to reading the front of the package)

In our first recipe we use pre-made spaghetti sauce which is fine if you learn to buy the "right" one. Finding the healthiest tomato sauce comes down to reading the nutrition label and making sure they have not added sugar to the item. All tomatoes contain sugar so the item will have sugar in it (that's unavoidable and fine as long as additional sugar has not been added, you can find that out by reading the nutrition label).

Here's an example:

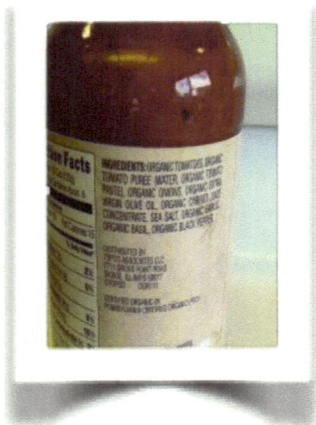

In reading the ingredients you can see that no sugar has been added making this a good choice. You can also understand what each ingredient is no "mystery" ingredients are science experiments here.

**Compare the label above to this label...**

And this would be a "bad" choice...This is not an ideal choice because sugar has been added, they are using soybean oil instead of a healthier option like Olive oil and it contains Yeast.

Just by comparing the two ingredients you can see which is the better choice. This is not an ideal choice because sugar has been added, they are using soybean oil instead of a healthier option like Olive oil and it contains Yeast.

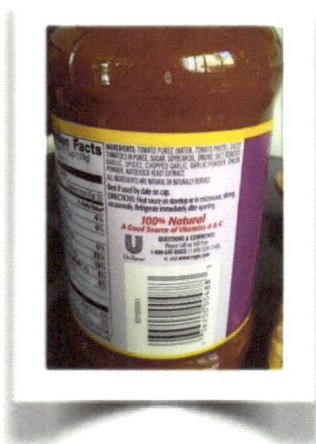

And both items were comparable in price!

Taking the time to read and understand nutrition labels is of paramount importance when it comes to optimum health and achieving your health and fitness goals!

Eat3691.com

Yes it takes a little extra time to read labels but think of it this way. If the food is in your 3-6-9 line up it means you are eating it regularly so it's worth the time to figure out what the best option is.

**Make this commitment to yourself here and now... "If it's going in my 3-6-9-1 line up I will know EXACTLY what it is I'm eating."**

Now let's take that statement for a test spin.
Do you have a coffee or sugary beverage in your 3-6-9-1 like a mocha or frilly morning pick me up drink?

I personally love coffee but I drink it with no sugar and about a tablespoon of real cream... (just a dash).

If you drink a syrupy coffee drink, or something similar to that, do you really know what's in it?

Remember the commitment you made to yourself a few sentences ago... If you're going to do something daily/weekly please learn what's in the foods you are consuming and make an educated decision about what you're putting in your body. Spend the time....you're worth it!

**Now it's time for Breakfast....**

## My Three Breakfasts-

The key with breakfast, for me, is I have learned to EAT IT!  When I was younger (and far less healthy) I used to skip breakfast.  Even as a kid, into teenage years, to young adult...  I hated breakfast and really enjoyed just grabbing a coffee instead but I turned the tables and learned to eat it.

If you want to be an athlete, or transform your body, you have to learn to eat consistently.. You have to fuel your body.

And not just athletes, for overall health and weight loss you have to learn to treat food as fuel.  This is so important because when you skip meals your metabolism gets to move in slow motion.  I know, I know we're tired of hearing about "metabolism" but if you're struggling with your weight and you're still skipping meals you need to hear it again.

Think of your metabolism like a fire.  You want to keep throwing small pieces of wood on that fire to keep it roaring all day.  Skipping meals is like failing to put wood on the fire and what happens then?  Poof!  It goes out!

Get that metabolism going by eating regularly (every 3 hours) and moving baby!
With this style of eating and implementing Strength training and cardio, into my life, I completely transformed my body and you can too.. ( I promise I wouldn't waste your time if I didn't know it could totally happen for you too!)

So the first key to breakfast is to eat it!

The second thing I want to mention about my 3-6-9  is timing is everything!
If you workout, early in the morning, drink a green smoothie (see recipe #1) within 30 minutes of completing your workout.  Then within 90 minutes of that eat a full meal.

If you start your day off, this way, you will begin see beautiful changes in your body very quickly.

My morning schedule looks like this:

**5:30-6:30am** Workout #1 of the day
**7am** - Green Smoothie
**8:30am** - Gallo pinto

and so on... I continue eating every 3 hours from that point on throughout the day. Stopping at about 7pm after dinner. I will typically have a cheese and cracker or small bite before bed but that's about it.

I cannot express enough how critical timing is for body transformation as well as athletic performance.

Get your timing down... and half the battle will have been won!

Now onto the recipes...

## Breakfast #1 Green Smoothies

I used to HATE fruit smoothies... I don't have much of a sweet tooth and have never been a huge, fruit, fan but I learned... literally taught myself, to drink these... because they make such a huge difference to your health and athletic performance.

For this recipe you'll need a high powered blender (like a Vitamix). This type of blender is worth the investment because they are powerful enough to make the smoothie.. smooth! and won't leave you with chewy chunks of leaves... Yuck!

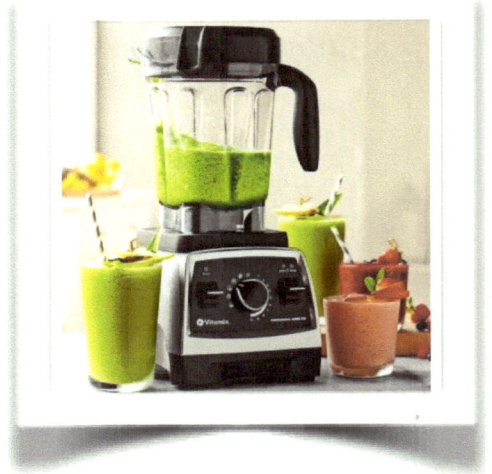

If you're new to green smoothies start out with spinach, as your greens, because most people find spinach is the most palatable and has the mildest flavor. Then you want to build up the quantity you put in there and variety of greens. Don't stay stuck on spinach.

If you can get you and your loved ones drinking green smoothies everyone's health will benefit!

Making Green Smoothies a part of your daily life will dramatically bring inflammation down in the body and as I'm sure you've heard by now. Inflammation is our number one health risk! Decreasing inflammation also speeds recovery time in athletes so again as far as a magic elixir this is it! I hope you learn to love them too!

## Basic starter recipe for green smoothies:

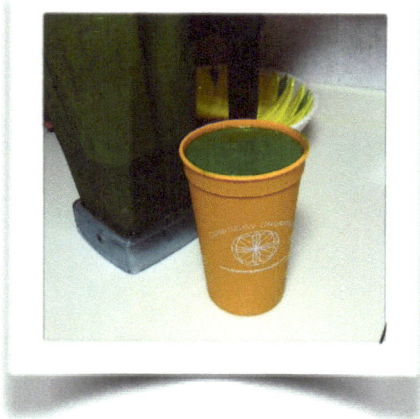

### Ingredients:
1 cup cold water
1 orange
1 banana
½ cup frozen blueberries
6 large handfuls of fresh spinach (or green of your choice ex: kale, swiss chard, red leaf lettuce, etc)

### Directions:
Blend the water and spinach, until it's liquid, and then add in the fruit and blend on high till smooth. Start with an 8 ounce serving and drink until full.

For an alternative, to this simple recipe, you can use any 3 pieces of fruit you like. As you get used to the taste you can also substitute the spinach with other types of healthy greens like kale and swiss chard. It's a great way to hide vegetables that you aren't too fond of, especially from your kids!

**Breakfast #2  Sunrise Breakfast Tacos**

I used to think I liked breakfast burritos until I went to Austin, Texas and had breakfast tacos.  Much less tortilla, makes it healthier, and they are delicious!

**Ingredients:**
2 corn tortillas
2 eggs
fresh mixed greens
fresh salsa
optional (left over chicken or ground turkey)

**Directions:** Scramble two eggs (I know you're supposed to add a little milk to your eggs as you scramble them but I personally do not drink milk and don't add anything to the eggs. I simply scramble them with a fork).  Spray a little non-stick Olive oil cooking spray in a small frying pan and heat the pan.  Pour the eggs into a hot frying pan and cook the eggs.

While that's going if I have left over ground turkey or chicken breast I will warm a serving of that in the microwave and then toss that into the eggs when they are nearly done.

Warm tortillas over the flame, of the stove, or toss in microwave for a few seconds.

Serve this topped with mixed greens and fresh salsa.

A delicious way to start the day!... Enjoy  (Serves 1)

# Breakfast #3 Gallo Pinto

This is one of my favorite high energy meals (I call it my secret weapon!) Apparently Gallo Pinto translates to Spotted Rooster which is kind of a fun name...

**To see a video of how we make Gallo go to www.EAT3691.com**

**Ingredients:**
1 medium onion chopped
2 green bell peppers chopped
1 cup of cooked Basmati or Jasmine rice
1 (30)oz can black beans (drained) or cook your own black beans

**Directions:** To make a large batch (enough for 3-4 servings) cook 1 cup of dry white rice according to instructions on rice.

In a separate pan stir fry the onion and green pepper in a bit of the liquid from your black beans. Cook until the onion is translucent. Add in the can of beans and cooked rice continuing stirring until heated thoroughly. After you get the basic recipe down you can play around with the spices and add cilantro, avocado, salsa, etc. (Serves 2-4)

For breakfast I typically eat mine with a fried egg on top. I also regularly have this meal over a bed of greens for lunch... Like I said it's a staple!

Eat3691.com

## Condiments and Spices I LOVE!

Before we go on any further I want to remind you that eating healthy, or being on a "diet" does not have to mean eating bland foods with no flavor!

Quite the opposite I find the more flavor I can add to my meals the more they satisfy.

So don't hold back when it comes to fresh herbs and dried spices.

Using things like:

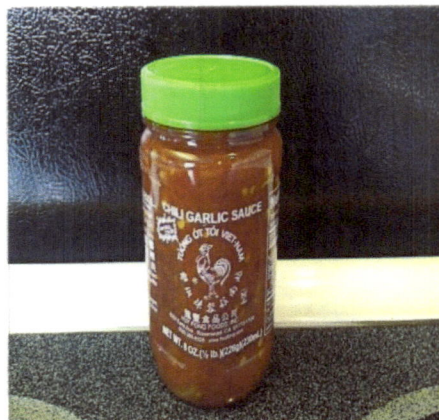

- Fresh Salsa

- lime, lemon

- garlic

- fresh herbs like basil, dill, thyme, etc.

- ground spices like turmeric, curry powder, paprika

I also like to pile on the chili's and the hot sauce. I know Sriracha is all the rage right now but I really like this sauce....

It's a Vietnamese chili garlic sauce it's hot, yummy and I can't live without it....I put it on everything! Don't forget to spice up your foods. If you satisfy your taste buds you won't be as tempted to over eat. The only reason you would need to watch out for some seasonings (like this) would be if you have high blood pressure. In some hot sauces you will find a high sodium content but for most people the amount of sodium you will get from adding something like this to a dinner, you make at home, is light years better than what you would get if you ate out at a restaurant. So if you cooked it at home.. SPICE IT UP....Baby!

**Step 3 still applies when it comes to condiments... Don't forget to read your labels!**

Eat3691.com

# My Six Lunches

As I mentioned, in the breakfast section, I eat every 3 hours but there is still a clear Breakfast, Lunch and Dinner, to my day, with the other 2-3 meals being more of a snack.  Snacks, for me, generally consist of items like:

* Triscuts (a shredded whole wheat cracker) with Turkey
* Turkey roll ups (2ozs of turkey breast with spinach, dill, or greens of some kind rolled up inside)
* Celery and salsa
* hard boiled eggs and veggies
* Triscuts and 1 oz of cheese (string or cheddar)
* an additional Green Smoothie (see breakfast #1)
* leftovers from one of my other 3-6-9's

The point here is I eat every 3 hours pretty religiously.  I started this back when I learned I was hypoglycemic and after fixing my diet and curing myself. I kept the habit because I just felt better eating that way.  It keeps that metabolism burning (remember?) and as an athlete, if you start skipping meals, you can feel the difference in your performance immediately... No Bueno!

Food is Fuel.  EAT! (just eat the right things ;-)

So for lunch I love to go out to eat... take a break... get away from the computer. Because of this I have specified how and what I order at a restaurant and separated those from lunches I eat at home.   I also love to get a good glass of Iced Tea... (unsweet please! Only the people from the South know what I mean by that.  It's how you order your tea without sugar here in the States.  Especially in the South they ask you "Sweet or Un-Sweet" and you better know what you like because it's a BIG difference.)

We haven't talked much about what we drink but I'll mention now... I drink a cup of coffee pretty much every day, a glass of ice tea several times a week.  Besides that it's water and sparkling water (plain, no artificial sweetener).  That's it  with the exception of beer and wine occasionally, never soda, never juice, never milk, never, ever, ever sports drinks like Gatorade.  Lots of water... We'll talk more about that in a later chapter.

# Lunch #1 Island Surprise Soup

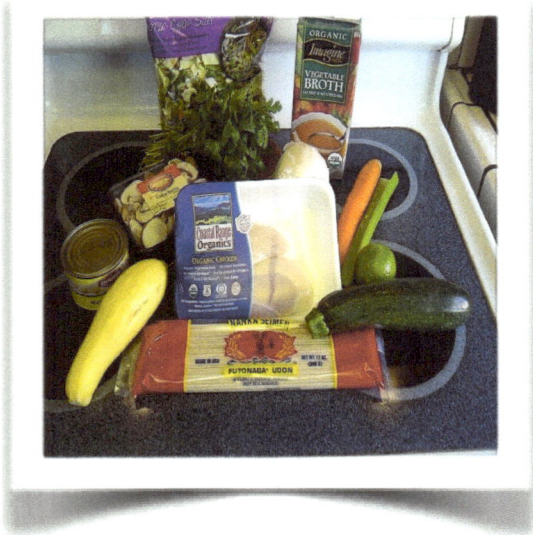

If I'm at a restaurant, like Olive Garden, I really enjoy soup and salad.  But If I'm at home my favorite soup to make is "Island Surprise".  We eat it quite often.  You could easily swap out the chicken for Tofu or shrimp if you like.

**Ingredients:**

1 stalk celery

1 carrot

½ a white onion

1-2 cloves garlic

1 zucchini

1 yellow squash

1 package of mushrooms

1 bag chopped Asian vegetables (or you can buy them separately napa cabbage, snow peas, bok choy are the most important)

1 bunch of Cilantro (use the whole bunch this really makes the dish)

1 (32oz.) container vegetable broth

1 can sliced water chestnuts

2  Chicken Breast

1 package of Udon noodles or Rice Noodles

1 tbsp of Basil

1 tsp black pepper

 juice of 1 lime

¼ cup of soy sauce

**Directions:** Start cooking the Chicken. I bring it to a boil, in a separate sauce pan and then let boil uncovered for 10 minutes. Then take it out and cut it into bite size chunks. Don't throw the water out though! Pour the water, the chicken was cooking in, and the pieces of Chicken into the soup pot. While you're waiting for the chicken to cook chop up the celery, carrot, onion and garlic and sauté them until soft, in a big soup pan. Once they've sautéed for a couple minutes pour in Vegetable broth, bring to a gentle boil and let simmer.

If your chicken is ready throw that in then Chop up the rest of the items (except for the noodles) and put them into the soup. Add 2 cups water and the rest of your seasonings, lime and soy sauce. Bring everything back to a boil then add in your noodles and boil for ten minutes. Simmer on low until you're ready to eat. Don't forget the hot sauce! (Serves 4)

# Lunch #2 Lettuce wraps and Sloppy Joe Boats

I really like lettuce wraps so I turn a bunch of stuff into lettuce wraps whether it be just grilling chicken and wrapping it in lettuce with a little hot sauce or making Sloppy Joe's without the bread.. or ordering my sandwich at a restaurant "wrapped" instead of on the bun (I find I actually prefer it in the lettuce.. try it you might like it!)

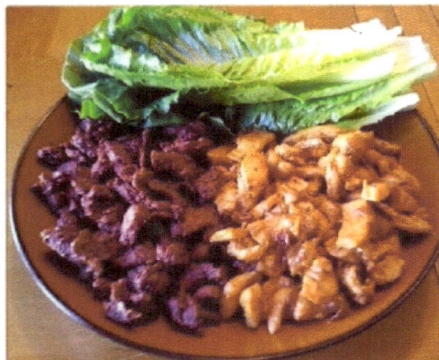

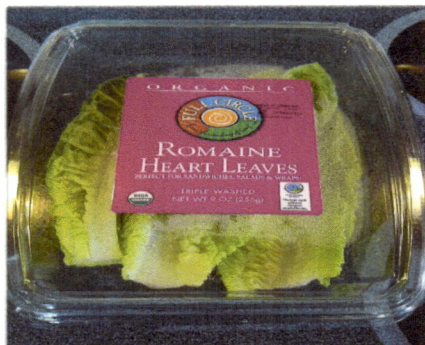

Below is our recipe for Sloppy Joe Boats and baked French fries

## Ingredients:

1lb ground turkey breast
pinch of black pepper
½ of a red onion chopped
1 (8oz) can of tomato sauce
½ cup ketchup (again not the healthiest choice but it adds just the right flavor)
¼ cup of bbq sauce
1 tsp chili powder
dash of hot sauce
Lettuce leaves
olive oil
chili powder
cayenne
1 small russet potato (per person)

**Directions:** Preheat the oven to 350 degrees. Wash and peel your potatoes and cut them into thin wedges, like French fries or fried potatoes, Take a cookie sheet and spray w/ a little olive oil cooking spray. Lay the potatoes out and drizzle w/ 2 tbsp olive oil then sprinkle w/ a little chili powder, cayenne pepper, and black pepper. With your hands mix them up a little so everything is coated evenly over the potatoes. Put them in the oven, keep an eye on them, and occasionally use a spatula to make sure they're not sticking. It will take about 40 minutes for them to cook, but as soon as they're tender and browning they're done.

Meanwhile- In a large skillet, brown the turkey, onion and black pepper until the turkey is no longer pink. You don't need to add any oil to do this, just keep an eye on it, and keep breaking it up. Stir in the tomato Sauce, ketchup, bbq sauce, chili powder, and hot sauce. Simmer this for about 10 minutes, stirring occasionally.

Serve this in a large bowl w/ the lettuce leaves on the side, so people can scoop out as much meat as they want to place in their lettuce leaves and serve the potatoes on the side. (Serves 2-4)

# Lunch #3 Turkey Burgers

We really don't eat beef, in our family (or at least very, very rarely as in a couple times a year). Although we think in moderation the Iron in beef and B12 adds to a healthy diet, due to factory farming and the conditions the animals are put through it is a moral choice, as well as a health choice. If you're not eating free range, grass fed, beef you are not doing your health any favors!

With that being said we eat a lot of free range turkey and chicken, so at our house burgers are made with ground turkey or ground chicken...and never with pre-made patties! Those are notoriously made with the worst parts of the animal and binders and yucky additives (Check your ingredient label and you'll see how much higher the fat content is in the pre-formed patties).

At a restaurant I will regularly order a grilled chicken breast sandwich or a Turkey Burger (lettuce wrap style). When I do this I know that the turkey is most likely 50% fat or higher so we don't eat them, at restaurants, as often as we make them at home.

**Ingredients:**

1lb Ground Turkey breast
Whole wheat buns or Lettuce for wraps
Tomato (sliced)
Onion (sliced)
Arugula
Sprouts
Dijon mustard

**Directions:** Season your meat with pepper and seasoning salt and form into patties. Grill on the BBQ or use your Foreman grill (another favorite tool around our house) ....and top with all the goodies listed above...The arugula and dijon mustard really help take this turkey burger over the edge with flavor! We typically serve this with steamed vegetables, our "vegified" pasta salad (see Lunch #4), or a side salad.

Often times I will add a kick to our burgers by dicing up mushrooms and spinach (very fine) and combining that into the patties, using an egg as binder, and seasoning with Garlic Powder and spices of your choice. This makes it feel like a whole new meal and the patties make great leftovers!... Yum! (Serves 2-4)

# Lunch #4 Pasta Salad that's been "vegified"

Pasta Salad is one of those things that can be really unhealthy or really healthy depending on how it's made.  Skip the mayo, use whole grain pasta and load it with veggies and you've got a decent meal.   Think of it more as a vegetable salad, with pasta in it, rather than a pasta salad with some vegetables in it and you'll be good to go.

### Ingredients:
1 box whole grain pasta
1 Cucumber (diced)
1 red bell pepper (diced)
Tomato (diced)
1 head of broccoli (chopped)
1 can kidney beans
¼ cup Italian dressing made with olive oil
1 tbsp Dijon mustard or ½ tsp ground mustard

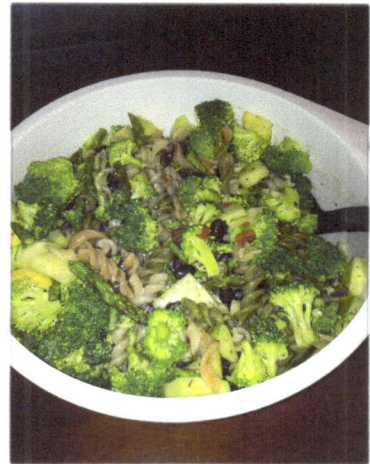

**Directions:**  While the pasta is cooking combine the dressing and mustard in a large bowl. Cut up the vegetables and toss them into the dressing mixture.  Drain the pasta and then I rinse it under cool water to help bring down the temperature a bit quicker.  Add the pasta to your vegetable mixture. Mix it all up and Refrigerate, when it's nice and cold taste it and if you need to add a little more dressing or leave the dressing out and let people add it to their taste.  (Serves 4)

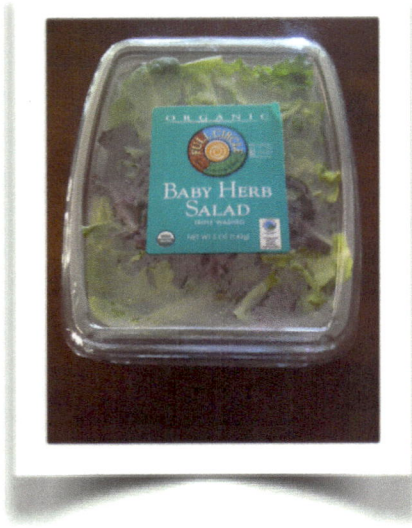

## Additional Recipe... And then of course there's always... "The Big salad"

It may sound boring but Yes it's definitely a staple in our house. "What do you want for lunch honey?.... How about a Big Salad? Okay sounds good!"

I buy a large variety of mixed greens for our salads including: Watercress, Dandelion root, Red leaf lettuce. At our grocery store they carry a pre-washed organic blend of lettuces called "Baby herb Salad" I love! It has all the mixed greens and dill and cilantro as well, that's what I generally use for the base of our Big Salads then just add in a variety of your favorite veggies.

### Ingredients:
Mixed greens
Cucumber
Red bell pepper
Broccoli
Sprouts
1 can kidney beans
Chopped turkey breast

**Directions:** Toss the lettuce in a big bowl and add in all of your chopped veggies... we also add in a can of drained kidney beans and some chopped turkey breast to make it more substantial. Our dressing of choice is typically bleu cheese (which has its health benefits in moderation) We also use Olive Oil based dressings or if you're really watching your diet...top with salsa instead.

## Lunch #5  Lentils and Quinoa on a bed of spinach or sautéed Greens

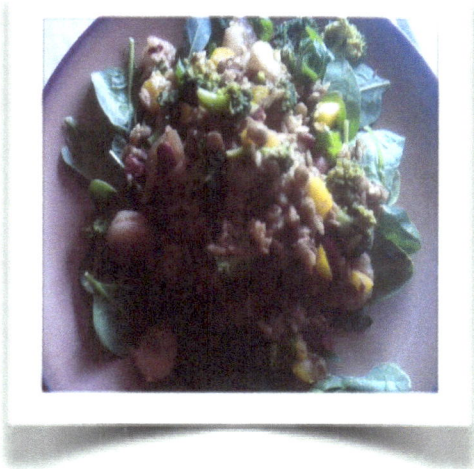

Quinoa and lentils are a main staple in our house. This is a meal we throw together with whatever seasonings we have on hand...typically some type of Curry flare is our favorite way of spicing it up and sometimes I add a can of stewed tomatoes.

### Ingredients:

1 cup cooked lentils
1 cup cooked brown rice or quinoa
1 head Broccoli
1 Yellow bell pepper
1 bunch Fresh spinach
1 Tsp Coriander
1Tbsp Turmeric
1 Tbsp Curry powder

**Directions:** Cook the lentils and Quinoa to the package specifications (or if I'm in a hurry I open a can of lentil soup and drain the liquid through a colander and add those instead of taking the time to cook the lentils).  When they're done put them in a large skillet with your chopped vegetables and spices.  Cook on medium heat until your vegetables get tender and then serve over a bed of fresh spinach.  (Serves 2-4)

Eat3691.com

## Just Sautéed Greens

I love sautéed spinach and kale!  Spinach cooks down much faster than kale but you can use the same ingredients for either one.  If you're not used to eating "greens" like these start with spinach and work up to Kale. Kale is a little stronger in flavor and can take some getting used to.

For this recipe you do need to use Olive Oil just be sure to measure.  A couple Tablespoons will do, to keep it from burning.

### Ingredients:
1 large bunch of kale or spinach (washed and chopped)
1 wedge of lemon or Tsp of Apple cider vinegar
 olive oil
Salt, pepper
fresh garlic.

**Directions:** Pour the olive oil in a large skillet.  Turn the heat to medium and add in your garlic, kale (or spinach), salt and pepper and a squeeze of lemon.  I find it easiest to use tongs to mix it all up and make sure the olive oil gets coated on everything. Cover and let steam for 10 minutes then uncover and keep cooking until tender. Again if you're using spinach this only takes about 5 minutes total.  Keep a close watch on your greens they can easily burn.

The recipe above is more of a curry flavor but we also use sautéed greens with Cumin seasoning as a bed for a healthy warm taco salad.  It's delicious!

**Another Great Fast Lunch or Dinner option** I do with sautéed greens is add them to a bowl of soup,  It makes for an easy meal to grab a can of minestrone or miso soup and add in a bunch of greens.  It's yummy and makes it a lot healthier! Simply toss the greens in as you warm the soup up and you're good to go!

**One more great thing to do with Kale is make Kale chips.**  Use the same ingredients above to make the recipe below.

**Directions for Kale chips:** Preheat oven to 425. Wash the kale and remove the bottom portion of the stalk. Tear the kale into palm size pieces and place them on a cookie sheet lined with tin foil. You can either combine the remaining ingredients in a bowl and pour the mixture over the kale or put them on separately by drizzling a small amount of olive oil over the leaves and then sprinkle the salt and pepper and squeeze a little lemon over it.

Then chop up the garlic and sprinkle it on. Take the leaves and flip them over and make sure they are all evenly coated. Bake for 12-14 minutes they will turn crispy like chips but you have to keep an eye on them because they do burn easily. Also be careful when you open the oven because the moisture from the Kale creates a lot of steam and it can come pouring out and surprise you! These are truly guiltless calories, if you monitor the amount of olive oil you use, so…. Enjoy!

Eat3691.com

# Lunch #6 Tuna Ceviche or What not to spill in your car...

This used to be one of my favorite "go to" meals to pack and take with me until the day the container opened and it spilled all over the floor of the car and in between the seats. Needless to say I had to immediately take the car to the detailers and luckily the smell didn't last long! It's still delicious though!

Whenever I get people to try this they're always surprised by how good it is. The key is you have to use all 6 limes (or at least close to it). The limes really make the difference!

**Ingredients:**
1 can tuna
6 limes
1 bunch cilantro (several sprigs, or to taste)
1 Serrano pepper (if you like spicy)
diced tomato
chopped white onion
Salt + Pepper

**Directions:** Take a can of tuna, drain, and put it in a bowl. Squeeze the juice of 6 limes, then add in; chopped cilantro, 1 chopped and seeded Serrano chili pepper, chopped tomato and diced white onion. Mix that all up and if you have time let it marinate in the refrigerator for a little while. (Serves 1-2)

This is good served with Triscuts (shredded whole wheat crackers), on celery, over a bed of lettuce or try something fun. This is a "Gorilla". I saw a gorilla for the first time at Whole Foods Market. It's a hollowed out cucumber and you use it as an edible vessel just like you would a sandwich.

To make a gorilla: Wash and but DO NOT PEEL the cucumber. Chop off the top ¼ of the cucumber and with an ice tea spoon or a melon baller hollow it out so all that remains is a little white on the inside. This is a "gorilla container".

Stuff your cucumber with the ceviche and enjoy!

## My Nine Dinners

I have no problem eating dinner... What I had to learn is to not make this my one and only HUGE meal of the day... I used to have the bad habit of skipping meals and end up starving by the end of the day. From about 3pm on I would want to eat everything in sight.

When I transformed my body that had to stop!

Now dinner for me is about the same size as the other meals in my day. Because I have fueled my body properly throughout the day I'm not starving by the time dinner rolls around and it's much easier to control cravings and make healthy choices.

I typically eat dinner around 6pm and am in bed by 9 (I also wake up daily at 4am) sleeping in for me is 6am. Again I'm giving you times because timing is important. I don't believe in the "don't eat before bed" story...

Fueling your body before bed is actually a good thing. A little protein or healthy fat.

But you can see how if someone is putting away a gallon of ice cream every night the "don't eat after 7pm rule" would be very helpful! It all comes down to your habits...

Dinners now may not be huge, like they used to be, but whenever possible I do prefer to sit down to a home cooked meal.

Here are the 9 dinners I eat the most often...

# Dinner #1 Healthier Potato Skins

I think it's silly potatoes get such a bad "rap" there are lots of healthy ways to stuff a potato and when you scoop out the vast majority of the inside of a potato, replace it with vegetables a (tiny amount) of cheese and bake it...you end up with a pretty healthy dish.  So who ever said you couldn't have healthy potato skins?

or if you're not watching your Carb consumption load the potato without losing any of the inside.  Like I said they shouldn't get a bad rap!  Just load em' up with healthy stuff...

**Ingredients:**

Russet potatoes 1-2 per person
Spinach
Broccoli
Chicken breast
Diced tomatoes
Cheese (any variety, tiny amount just for flavor)

This is a basic recipe any vegetables that sound good can go in there...beans are great too.  Sometimes we do a BBQ version with chicken breast, kale broccoli and corn.... sometimes Mexican style with ground turkey, black beans, spinach and salsa.

**Directions:**  Preheat your oven to 350.  Wash your potatoes then poke a couple holes in them with a fork.  Bake the potatoes at 350 degrees for about 45 minutes or until they are tender (if you are cooking more than 4 potatoes you will have to extend the cooking time by 15 minutes).  While they're baking chop up your vegetables and cook your chicken breast.  You can bake the chicken at the same time in the oven alongside the potatoes or you can grill it.

When the potatoes are ready take them out of the oven and very carefully cut them in half (they will be very hot so this part is tricky) scoop out the center of the potato leaving the skin completely intact.  Place them on a cookie sheet covered in foil and start spooning in your toppings (broccoli, chopped chicken, tomatoes, spinach, finish with a little bit of cheese).

Put them back in the oven for another 10 minutes and serve!

# Dinner #2 Sweet & Spicy Shrimp (this is yummy, but spicy)

**Ingredients:**

1lb shrimp (serves 2-4)

1 ½ tsp cornstarch

pinch of white or black pepper

¼ chicken broth

¼ cup ketchup (*I know not very healthy but sometimes it adds just the right flavor!*)

2 tbsp low sodium soy sauce

2 tbsp rice vinegar

2 tbsp chili garlic sauce

2 tsp olive oil

6 cloves chopped garlic

1 tsp fresh ginger grated

1 shallot chopped

1 jalapeno seeded and chopped

¼ cup egg white

Jasmine rice

You will also need 1 package of edamame (for optional side dish)

**Directions:** Thaw your shrimp according to package instructions or you can use raw, peeled and deveined, shrimp for this one. In a bowl combine the cornstarch and white or black pepper then coat your shrimp. Set aside.

Cook your rice according to instructions

Cook your edamame according to package instructions (usually takes about 2 minutes) and then set aside.

In a bowl combine chicken broth, ketchup, soy sauce, rice vinegar and chili garlic sauce; set aside.

Heat oil in a skillet or wok, over high heat. Add garlic, ginger, shallot and jalapeno stir it for about 30 seconds then add in the shrimp and cook for about 2 minutes. Then slowly pour the egg white over the shrimp and continue to cook and stir for another 30 seconds. Serve over rice.

Don't forget your edamame serve as a yummy side dish!

# Dinner #3 Throw it together...Turkey Chili

This is a great "go to" dinner. It's simple to throw together and because most of the ingredients are canned it's easy to have everything on hand. Below are the spices I use when I have time.. if I don't I'll grab a packet of pre-mixed chili spices from the grocery store.

**Ingredients:**

1lb ground turkey breast
1 cup red pepper, chopped
1 can kidney beans
1 can chili beans
1 onion, chopped
1 tsp paprika
1 tsp ground cumin

1/8 tsp ground cayenne pepper
1 can diced tomatoes in juice
1 can tomato sauce
1 clove garlic, minced
2 tsp chili powder
1 bay leaf
Salt and pepper to taste

**Directions:** In a large soup pot, brown your turkey on medium to high heat. Season with the salt and pepper. Cook for 3 to 5 minutes, breaking up the turkey into pieces, until browned all over. Reduce the heat to low, and add the peppers, onion and garlic powder, paprika, cumin and cayenne pepper. Cook, stirring for 1 minute. Increase the heat to medium, and add the tomatoes, tomato sauce, beans and bay leaf. Bring to a boil over high heat. Reduce the heat to medium-low and simmer for 15 minutes, uncovered. It's ready when you are...remember to remove the bay leaf before serving (or make it a game, whoever finds it in their bowl, doesn't have to help with the dishes). (Serves 4)

Eat3691.com

# Dinner #4 Moore Please

My maiden name is Moore and this comes from something my mom used to throw together and we somehow started referring to it as "Moore" in our family...It has become a comfort food and staple in our home.

**Ingredients:**
1lb ground turkey breast
1 large can diced or stewed tomatoes (read the ingredients nothing added just tomatoes)
1 can plain tomato sauce (nothing added just tomatoes)
Fresh or dried basil
Dried Oregano
Salt & Pepper
Fresh garlic or garlic powder
1 box or bag whole grain pasta (any shape you like)
1 red bell pepper (diced)
1 bunch fresh spinach
1 zucchini (diced)
½ white onion (diced)
Mushrooms

**Directions:** Season the turkey with a little salt and pepper and brown it with the onions (no need to add oil just keep your eye on it). While that's cooking get the water for your pasta boiling and dice the vegetables. When the meat is ready add in the can of tomatoes and sauce and then season with basil, oregano and garlic to taste. Add in all your chopped veggies, cover and let simmer while your pasta cooks. When the pasta is ready drain the water and toss the meat and vegetable mixture over the noodles and mix it all up...that's Moore! (Serves 4)

Eat3691.com

# additional recipe ... Spaghetti with Vegetables

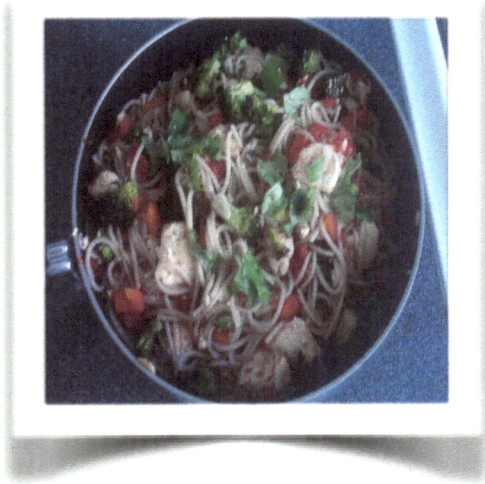

I'm not afraid of pasta but as you see when I eat it. It's not a heaping plate of noodles with sauce on top. It's an almost equal ratio vegetables to pasta.

## Ingredients:

1 pkg whole grain spaghetti
Broccoli
Fresh basil
Red bell pepper
Mushrooms

Cauliflower
Zucchini
Yellow summer squash
Olive oil
Fresh garlic

**Directions:** Get your pasta cooking and while that's cooking chop all your veggies. Sauté them in a large skillet with a couple tablespoons of olive oil and Fresh garlic. Drain the spaghetti and put it back in your pot and toss your vegetable mixture over the pasta. Serve with fresh basil on top, a little Parmesan cheese and of course...Hot sauce!

# Dinner # 5  No... No... No... Lasagna

This Lasagna contains no cheese and no noodles but it's so good you won't even miss them! When my husband made this for me the first time I was floored!  I could not believe how good it was and now I prefer it to conventional lasagna.

### Ingredients:
1  eggplant, cut lengthwise in ¼ inch slices to resemble lasagna noodles
1 zucchini, cut lengthwise in ¼ inch slices
1 pkg ground turkey breast meat
1 jar Marinara sauce **(no sugar added, rule #3) **
1 tsp chopped fresh basil or dried basil
Pinch freshly ground black pepper
Pinch cayenne pepper
¼ tsp ground coriander

**Directions:** Preheat oven to 400 degrees F
Lightly coat a nonstick cookie sheet with cooking spray.  Lay eggplant and zucchini slices on the sheet, cover with foil, and bake for about 15 minutes or until slices are soft.  Remove from the oven and set aside.

Place ground turkey, coriander, black pepper and cayenne pepper in the skillet and sauté until brown- approximately 3 to 4 minutes.  *Important Note* You will see throughout this book that I use the word "sauté" loosely.  When I say it I mean to put it in a skillet with no oil unless otherwise noted.  Never add oil if at all necessary.  One tablespoon of olive oil adds 120 calories to your meal so even though it's a healthy fat it can still quickly make you fat!  When I add oil it is explicitly written.

Lasagna assembly; Lightly spray an ovenproof baking dish with cooking spray.  Alternate layers of baked eggplant, ground turkey, marinara and baked zucchini.  Top w/ marinara sauce.  Repeat the process if you still have room.

Bake for 15-20 minutes or until heated thoroughly.  Top w/ chopped fresh basil and Enjoy! (Serves 2-4)

# Dinner #6 Red Cabbage Tostadas

We eat A LOT of Mexican food… Substituting red/purple cabbage leaves in place of tortillas is a great way to make dinner more fun and healthier. Call them "Purple Tacos" and maybe the kids will even be more willing to try!

**Ingredients:**
1 head of purple cabbage
½ of a chopped onion
1lb ground turkey breast or free range ground beef, bison or meat of your choice
Fresh guacamole
Fresh salsa
Chopped tomatoes
1 pkg Taco seasoning

**Directions:** Begin browning your turkey and add in the taco seasoning and chopped onion, cook thoroughly.

While that's cooking wash your cabbage (do your best to keep the leaves whole) and pat them dry.

Put all the ingredients in an assembly line fashion and have everybody assemble their own, this way if you like more or less of something you can alter it to your taste. Have ingredients like cheese and sour cream as options or eliminate them all together. (Serves 2-4)

I pretty much live on fresh salsa… I snack on it with celery sticks (and tortilla chips), I use it to top baked potatoes, salads and pretty much eat it every day. I'm not going to provide a recipe for it though because although I like my homemade salsa I know I don't make it correctly and I never serve it to guests. It's pretty much just tomatoes, cilantro, serrano pepper, jalapeno, onion and a little salt, pepper and lime thrown in my Vita Mix. I like it but like I said it's not "guest quality" so with that being said what I usually do is buy a good store bought fresh salsa. There are some great quality fresh salsas in grocery stores around here so no need to bust my butt let the pro's do it!

Eat3691.com

# Dinner #7 Shrimp Cocktail Meal

Otherwise known as what I order if we go to red lobster w/ baked potato (no salt) and side salad...tell them not to bring the biscuits to the table :-)

**Ingredients:**
1/2 lb Shrimp (fresh, uncooked)
Cocktail sauce
1 russet potato
1 head broccoli

**Directions:** Boil water. While that's boiling clean and de-vein shrimp. Pour uncooked shrimp in boiling water and remove from heat. Pour into strainer in 3 minutes. Refrigerate shrimp w/crushed ice. While that's cooling bake the potato and steam your broccoli. Serve with cocktail sauce and a squeeze of lemon. (Serves 1-2)

## additional recipe... My Shrimp Bowl

I also have a strange recipe I throw together at home with frozen shrimp.

**Ingredients:**
White rice
finely chopped vegetable mixture (radishes, broccoli, red bell pepper, celery, cucumber)
Sea vegetables( if you can get them) or dried Sea weed flakes (dulce)
defrosted Cooked Shrimp

**Directions:** I cook the rice according to package specifications and while that's cooking defrost my shrimp and chop the veggies. When the rice is ready I toss the shrimp in a pan just to warm it up a bit.

I do not cook the vegetables at all. I leave them raw. Place the rice in a bowl and top with chopped veggies and shrimp, a touch of sea weed (dulce) or sea vegetables if you were able to find some for flavor, hot sauce and soy sauce and voi la! I have a delicious Sushi Bowl at home!

Eat3691.com

## Dinner #8  Spaghetti Squash or Where's the noodles? .... Spaghetti

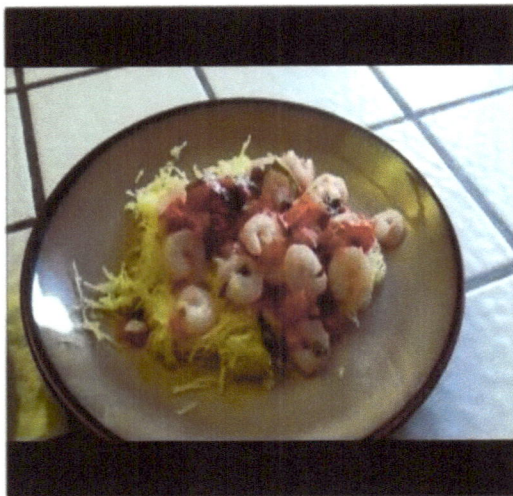

Throw a wrench in your typical spaghetti night and serve spaghetti without the noodles.  The first time you make this meal I recommend making spaghetti the way you normally do and simply switching out the noodles with spaghetti squash. Or you can ease yourself, and those you're cooking for, into it by doing half pasta, half squash but after awhile you may be surprised to find you start to prefer it this way.  I know I do! ... For a video on how to cook spaghetti squash go to www.EAT3691.com

### Ingredients:

1 jar of  Marinara Sauce (remember our rule #3 :-)

1 spaghetti squash
Fresh basil and garlic

**Directions:** Prepare the Spaghetti squash using the instructions below.  While that's cooking warm up your marinara.  Once your squash is ready, plate it and cover with sauce.  Enjoy! (Serves 2-3)

This is what a spaghetti squash looks like. They are very easy to make just quarter the squash and spoon out the seeds and stringy bits (like you would a pumpkin) You will be left with a nice smooth surface about 1-2 inches thick of squash. Place it flesh down into a microwave safe dish in about 1 inch of water.  Cook for 10 minutes.  It is now ready to shred.  Take a fork and run it along the inside of the flesh and you will see it magically turn into long noodle like pieces...very cool!

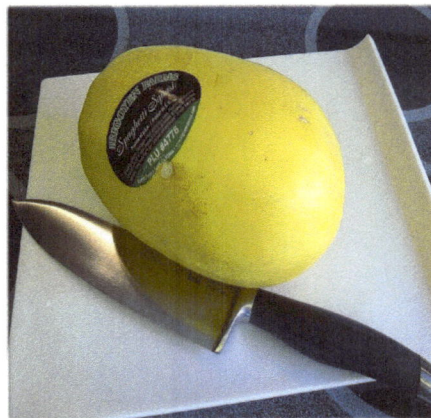

# Dinner #9 Not so Fried Rice

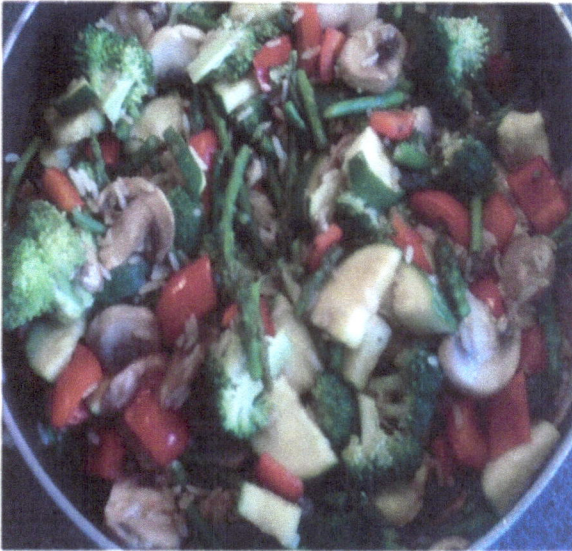

Along the same line as pasta salad this can either be made very healthy or completely the opposite. To make a healthy version think of it more along the lines of steamed vegetables with rice, added, rather than steamed rice with a couple vegetables tossed in. When you look down at your plate you should see a ton of veggies with speckles of rice.

**Ingredients:**

1 pkg boil in a bag brown rice or brown rice (yields 2 cups)
1 head broccoli (chopped)
1 bundle asparagus (chopped)
1 red bell pepper (chopped)
2 cloves garlic
Bok choy (chopped)

1 carrot (grated)
6-12 snow peas
1 container mushrooms
1 tsp grated fresh ginger
Soy sauce to taste

**Directions:** Cook the rice and while it's cooking Sauté the veggies in a large skillet or Wok, with garlic, soy sauce and ginger (no oil needed for cooking if you just keep an eye on it). As soon as the vegetables are beginning to tender turn them off and wait for the rice to be done (you don't want them over cooked and mushy). When the rice is ready add it to the vegetables. Again you want your ratio of vegetables to rice to be completely the opposite of what you're used to seeing....so don't add too much rice. Add soy sauce and hot sauce to taste when you serve. (Serves 4)

Eat3691.com

# Dessert

I'm not a huge dessert fan, by any means, but if it's chocolate on top of chocolate with chocolate drizzled over it I'll probably love it!  If you are the type of person (like my husband) who craves dessert regularly.  Then I would recommend two things:
First- sugar is very unhealthy and it's important for your 3-6-9 you detox from your processed sugar addiction completely.  Contact us for cleanses if you need help or don't just want to go cold turkey...

There is no place for processed sugars in a healthy 3-6-9-1 (except on Cheat day of course)  Every now and then no problem but first you need to break the addiction.  Second- cravings (especially for sugar) are a way of the body signaling you it's not getting the nutrition it needs.  Your body is so smart it knows the fastest, simplest way to take in energy is with sugary foods and drinks, including alcohol.  Until you give your body what it needs and detox from the sugar addiction your cravings will remain something willpower alone cannot compete with.

So take your sugar cravings seriously.  It's a signal and it's time to listen to what your body is trying to tell you.

When all this is in balance, you'll still enjoy treats but you won't NEED them.. make sense?

Just a bite will do and that's pretty much what my 1 dessert comes down to

If I want a treat I have the best.  A couple bites of the best chocolate and I'm set.
I really don't indulge in desserts more than once a month, not because I'm trying to restrict myself simply because I don't crave it.

But let's say you just really enjoy your sweets.. That's fantastic.  Whole fruit Smoothies and whole fruit combinations should suit you well.

Here is a recipe that will make most chocolate lovers swoon and it's REALLY healthy... Enjoy!

## Banana Sundae
Serves 1-2

### Ingredients:
3 bananas
2 Medjool dates
Raw cacao powder.

Take 2 ½ bananas and chop them up into bite size slices. Keep the remaining half of a banana and throw it into your blender with 2 pitted dates and 1 Teaspoon of cacao powder, blend with just enough water to make it a thick sauce. Pour that over the sliced bananas and enjoy!

## Chocolate Smoothie

Bananas and Cacao powder (and cacao nibs) make the most delicious chocolate smoothies... Use water or coconut water and blend 4 bananas with 1-2 Tbsp Cacao powder or nibs and you'll think you're cheating but you're not!

You can also freeze this for a delicious ice cream treat.

# Water...

As an athlete you learn real quickly not having enough water will mean poor performance but in our everyday lives it's easy not to notice that lethargic feeling creeping in.  We rarely attribute that sluggishness to not having enough water but it affects so much of our health.

We know water is crucial to our very survival.  Next to oxygen, water is the most essential element to human life; the body usually cannot survive longer than 3 days without water (a maximum of 1 week). Water is essential to the functioning of every single cell and organ system in the human body.

The funny part is even though we know that, even though we've had that drilled into our heads from the time we were born...we still don't drink even close to enough of it every day!

We've all had the 8 glasses 8ounces drilled into our heads which is quite humorous... so what you're telling me is that my 200lb husband and I (at 130....okay make that 135 most days) require the same amount?  That's asinine! That's like saying your car requires the same amount of fuel whether you go 100 miles or 1000 miles.  Nope the bigger you are the more you need.  The fact of the matter is most dietitians recommend this formula when determining your daily water quota

.66 x your weight in pounds = ounces you need per day

Multiply your weight in pounds by the number .66 and you have the amount in ounces you need every day.  For example the equation for me would look like this .66 x 135 = 89.1 ounces a day (well above the widely talked about 64 oz. recommendation and I'm light!)

This is the formula I have adhered to as my minimum and I can tell when I don't get it!  A reduction of 4-5% in body water can result in a 20-30% decrease in work and exercise performance.

Most sports nutritionists and trainers will tell you not to include the water you drink during a workout in your daily requirement. What you drink during a workout does not count towards your daily total. The fluids you consume during a workout are lost, as you sweat, so they don't count! And if you're curious the general recommendation for amounts to drink during a workout is 4 ounces. every 15 minutes (in mild weather in humid conditions the amounts may be as much as doubled). So you need to consume one of those 16.9 ounce bottles of water during your workout...at a minimum! Keep in mind 4oz is a generalization just like the magic "64 oz" number so take into consideration your size, the intensity of the workout and if you're really pushing yourself or not feeling good during your workouts talk to a Sports nutritionist and find out what YOU need.

My husband, Tony, has been drinking basically nothing but water since the day we met. He occasionally has an ice tea or root beer (as in a couple times a year) but that's it...he drinks water, no milk, no alcohol, no juice, no soda and he's one of the healthiest people I've ever met. When we first got together I was shocked by how much water he drank (not so much that it was all he drank) but by the amounts, the volume. We have to battle with servers to bring us a pitcher or a couple glasses of water so they don't have to keep coming over to our table because they're so not used to seeing that.

Getting yourself and everyone else in the family to reach for water instead of soda, juice or a sports drink may seem tough but believe it or not once you get off of the sugary drinks you will appreciate the more subtle taste of water.

Take your frozen fruit and add a couple pieces to a glass of water instead of ice cubes. Try it...it makes your water a lot more fun and tasty!

We keep a pitcher of water in the fridge at all times with fresh or frozen fruit in it... think outside the box you're not just limited to a slice of lemon.

Try strawberries, oranges, limes, pineapple, apple, frozen blueberries
mint, basil, cucumber

Eliminating sugary drinks (including juice) is a great start for improving the overall health of your family....

From our family to yours...Cheers!

# Exercise and Move!

Movement is crucial to a healthy body. Studies now indicate the more you move the better for your health. The old guidelines of 30 minutes a day 3 days a week is simply not going to cut it!

You have to move!

We have set up a membership into our Online Workout Community just for you!

If you have read this far we want to help you take the next step, so email us at

OnlineWorkouts@Eat3691.com

And we will get you started right away!

# Fueling your body during a workout

Whether it's sports drinks, protein bars, Gu Shots or powders I find there is a lot of confusing information, out there, about what you should consume pre-workout, post-workout and during your workout and to put it bluntly you're being sold a bunch of malarkey and expensive pee!

If you're workouts consist of an hour or so at the gym each day, then you may not concern yourself with your "workout fuel' just having a healthy 3-6-9 will suffice but when you start increasing your training, for longer endurance events; like your first marathon or triathlon or taking whatever sport you're in to the next level, then the fuel you take in during your workouts becomes very important.

When I initially started doing endurance races I spent loads of money on expensive "recovery" powders with fancy names, promising wonders, but I quickly learned the same is true for every day diet as it is for fueling your workouts...

Eat things that grow that way in Nature! If it exists in Nature your body will have an easier time absorbing it and ultimately getting fuel out of it.

If it's made in a factory it's going to be a lot harder for your body to break down and end up taxing your energy system instead of giving you energy! When I switched from Gu shots (a sugary gu substance made with high fructose corn syrup, regularly handed out at marathons and other sporting events) to Medjool Dates during my workouts I could tell the difference immediately and never looked back.

Now if I eat a Gu shot or Power block or any of those processed "energy" products they make me sick. My fuel of choice now... Green smoothies post workout and Dates or sweet potatoes during and a healthy 3-6-9 the rest of the time. I eat two dates every hour of workout. So if it's a two hour run I would eat 4 dates... and water.

The simplest purest foods will react the best in your body and give you the most fuel.

Give it a try! You'll love the results. Speaking of results...

## Results you should expect to see

As you begin following a new 3.6.9.1 you will begin to notice looser fitting clothing and changes to your body within the first few days.  Congrats on that!  It's really important you, take time to, notice those changes and acknowledge what a great job you're doing.  It's always amazing to me how quickly the body changes, when we allow it.  THE POWER OF THE BODY TO HEAL AND TRANSFORM IS AMAZING...

Use those subtle changes to inspire you and motivate you into the following week.

If you don't celebrate these little changes you'll find yourself stuck waiting for a BIG change and <u>that's not how the body works</u>... it's step by step, one inch here, one inch there, and before you know it you've arrived at the BIG change but by then you're used to it because it happened so gradually.  Make sense?

So if you don't celebrate, or at least acknowledge the little stuff, you may give up quickly because you're waiting for something that just doesn't come that way.

Here are some ways to tune in to the changes you are accomplishing:

* You may notice you're sleeping better
* Moods are more even and happier
* Your clothes fit better
* Skin lookers healthier and brighter
* People begin asking "What are you doing you look different.  Did you lose weight?"
* You may notice fewer aches and pains throughout your body
* Faster recovery after workouts
* Less maniacal cravings (more control)
* More energy for workouts and inspiration to GOYA

Take note of all of this.  If you really want to get into it, journal these things down, along with your diet and exercise.  We call it a "Positive Proof Journal".  Keeping this type of journal gives your brain something to build upon so when you start to feel like giving up, or you start trying to convince yourself things aren't changing, you can go back and remind yourself where you really came from.

Again because the change happens so subtly you will start to get used to the new lightness you feel, very quickly, and there will come a week where you won't have that big hit of "Wow I can really tell this is working" and that's when you need to remind yourself how much is different...and that's when your *Positive Proof Journal* will really come in handy.

**Now let's talk measurements:**

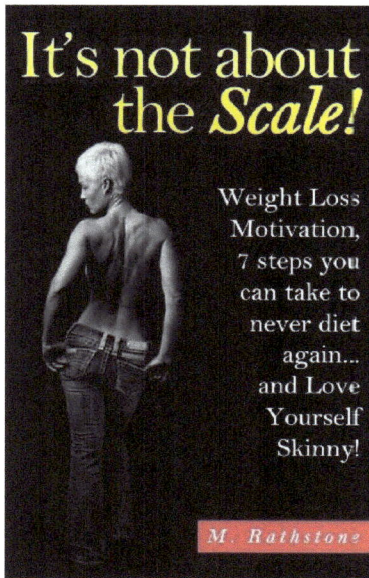

I pick on scales a lot... See my book *Its Not about the Scale*

but if you use one don't be embarrassed about it. If you use it to confirm what you can already tell is going on in your body, fine.  If you get on it guessing (and hoping) as to what it's going to say, then seriously reach out to me because it means you really aren't getting how the body works yet and that's important to us.

If you own a scale you will want to weigh yourself on Friday and Monday mornings only (it's really, really unproductive to weigh yourself daily).

If you're like most people you will weigh the least on Friday mornings and the most on Mondays (we always have to weigh at the same time of day, first thing in the morning, otherwise it really becomes even more of a useless tool for the home).  Don't freak out about your weight climbing up a bit since Friday, it's going to happen.

**Plus we recommend one cheat day a week where you allow yourself to eat absolutely anything you've been craving.**

One final thing on scales... Would you rather weigh 140lbs and have a tight, toned, healthy body, with loads of energy, to work out, and get through your day?
Or
Weigh 110lbs flappy skin, still embarrassed to be in a bikini, sick and with no energy... But you've got the #....?

I know the numbers would be different for everyone but you get the picture I'm after. It's a legitimate question because there are some people out there who really do want the bragging rights of the number (it's not my job to tell you what your goals should be) so if that's what you want. I can tell you how to get there so be real with yourself and what it is you want to accomplish or you could be wasting your time with this program.

This program is going to give you the tight, toned, energetic, healthy body. So if you're ready to proceed... YAY!

Here are some more telling ways of measuring:

- Take Before pictures. Front/both sides/ Back in a bathing suit or at least tight top and shorts.
- The next powerful tool is measurements. If you have a tape measure go ahead and pick a couple places to measure, hips, stomach, chest. And write those down in your positive proof journal.
- Finally your clothes are the best measuring tool you've got. So pick an outfit which is too tight, right now, and use that as more proof. Step into it each week and see how different it fits by the end!

Measure and retake photos once a month...

Transformation is absolutely within your grasp!

Eat like us, move like us and you will amaze yourself by creating your own...

**Be-YOU-ti-ful 3,6,9,1!**

See the rest of our series coming soon:

3-6-9-1 For Runners

3-6-9-1 Goes Raw

3-6-9-1 on a Budget

3-6-9-1 for vegetarians

3-6-9-1 on the go!

3-6-9-1 for the Fitness Enthusiast

Thanks for joining us...

Molli Rathstone

P.s. Think you have a Super healthy 3-6-9-1 you'd like to share with the world? Email us.... we'd love to see it and get you in the next book of the series!
***Staff@Eat3691.com***

www.ingramcontent.com/pod-product-compliance
Lightning Source LLC
Chambersburg PA
CBHW060817270326
41930CB00002B/70